Beside the Still Waters

Having Faith Even When.......

Rev. Dr. A'Shellarien D. Anthony-Lang

Jesse Hammond,

May This Book Bless Your Life

Love

[signature]

Beside the Still Waters
Copyright © 2012 by Rev. Dr. A'Shellarien Anthony-Lang

Desakajo Publishing
Wilmington, DE
www.desakajosflo.com

Dedication

This book is dedicated to my son, Baby Corey (11/11/99-11/11/99) for I have learned to live with losing you while at the same time miss you every day.

Table of Contents

Introduction

"The Lord is my Shepherd I shall not want"

Have you ever wondered how you were going to live without someone you love? Has the very thought of waking up without them or going to bed without them haunted your thoughts? I often wondered how people survive after someone very close to them dies. I could not imagine what it would be like and had no desire to find out. I had people that I knew die even family members but they were not close to me. I had the unfortunate experience of losing my son. It was unexpected, I was unprepared, and the whole experience was unbelievable. I remember it like it was yesterday. I was 39 weeks pregnant with my third child and second son. It was a Wednesday evening and something did not feel right so I called my midwife to share my concern. The office told me to just wait until morning because I had an early appointment the next day. I went to sleep that night feeling unsure but trusting the midwife.

Thursday morning I woke up as I always do and kissed my five year old son, K'Aelle and two year old daughter, Cache'. My husband stayed home with our children and I left for my appointment with the expectation that everything would be fine. When I got there the nurse asked me how things were going and I shared that I had called the night before because something did not feel right. She took out the heart monitor to listen to my son's heartbeat and could not find it. She acted like it was nothing and went to find the doctor. The doctor tried as well and could not find my son's heartbeat either. They looked at each other with horror in their eyes yet attempted to be very calm with me and shared that they were sending me upstairs for an ultrasound. At this point my faith was saying this is just a mistake so I will not worry. God would not allow this to happen to me, right?

I went upstairs and waited in the hallway for a room and eventually had an ultrasound. The technician did the ultrasound and would not share what she did or did not see. She rushed out to get another technician. The next technician performed a second ultrasound and looked at the first technician in horror and they calmly told me that they needed to go get the doctor. The doctor came in and performed a third ultrasound and looked at me with sadness and said, "We cannot find your baby's heartbeat, we believe that he has died." I was speechless. I could not believe that God would allow this to happen to me. I cried more in that moment than I cried in my whole life. I called my husband and told him and he was speechless as well. He attempted to console me and reassure me that it was not my fault and that God knew what God was doing.

Honestly, I did not want to hear that right then because I was angry. How could God allow this to happen to ME? I was doing my best to live right, love people, and serve God the best I knew how. While I was wrestling with my faith the doctor tells me that I have to deliver the baby and that they were going to induce my labor. So not only has my baby died now I have to go through labor to only go home empty handed. I was lying on the table talking to God while my husband was on his way. I had some questions that I needed answers to. Why? Why me? Why now? Why this way? What did I do wrong? Is this a test? My faith was shaken, my hope was devastated, and my future was forever changed. My heart was broken and nothing could change that, now what?

My husband arrived and labor began. It lasted four hours and I can remember secretly believing that God could turn this whole thing around. I recalled the miracles of Jesus and said surely God is still in the miracle working business and there is a chance that my baby will be born alive. It was finally time to push and he came out with one push and I caught him in my hand because the doctors had stepped out of the room. I listened for a cry and heard nothing. The nurses cleaned him up put clothes on him and asked me if I wanted to see him. I had to see if my miracle happened. I had secretly told God that if he allowed my baby to live I would……. My son was not breathing, there was no life, and there was no miracle for me that day. I looked at him and saw that he was a beautiful baby with big hands and feet. He was cute. I wondered what color his eyes were, what his cry would have sounded like, whether he would have smiled at me like my first son, K'Aelle. I handed him back to the nurse and felt empty.

The medicine that the doctor gave me made me very weak. I could not do anything, I could not sit up, feed myself, go to the bathroom or anything. My husband stayed with me all night to take care of me and I am forever grateful to him for that. I remember feeling so lost. I felt like I was in the twilight zone. It was so unreal. I remember wondering where God was in the midst of my pain. I wondered how I was going to leave the hospital without my son. How was I going to go on without him? In the midst of that thought something told me to call my house and check my messages. The message that I heard changed my life forever. My husband's best friend from Atlanta called my phone and began to sing "*Jesus you're the center of my joy. All that's good and perfect comes from you. You're the heart of my contentment, hope for all I do. Jesus you're the center of my joy. When I've lost my direction, you're the compass for my way. You're the fire and light when nights are long and cold. In sadness, you're the laughter that shatters all my fears. When I'm all alone your hand is there to hold. Jesus you're the center of my joy. All that's good and perfect comes from you. You're the heart of my contentment hope for all I do. Jesus you're the center of my joy*". He did not say anything he just sang. I knew it was God because he had no idea that our son died. I played that song at least ten times and cried and cried and cried. It was in those moments that my faith shifted. Although I was devastated I began to feel God's presence and accept that God had been with me the whole time. Baby Corey was with God and in a much better place than I was. When I quieted the voices long enough to hear God's voice God shared with me that had my son lived he would have been miserable. I had toxemia and my son was not getting the oxygen and the nutrients that he needed throughout his time in my womb. The only way for Baby Corey to be the healthy and happy baby that I asked God for was for God to take him home. It hurt but I understood. God was my Shepherd and I had allowed my pain to cause me to distance myself from my Shepherd. God never left me, I temporarily left God. Unfortunately as we walk through our grief, we may walk away from God, temporarily. Does that mean we have no faith? Does it mean that God won't be there when we return? Does it mean that God does not understand? No, No, and No. God is so much more loving than we could ever imagine. God is so much more compassionate than we could ever dream.

As I grieved the loss of my son I had to realize that prayer, talking to God, helped to soothe my pain. The very motion of stilling myself long enough to feel God with me changed my life. When I was eight I was a member of an African American Synagogue in Harlem, NY. I learned a prayer called Mode Ani. In the Hebrew faith tradition prayer is a lifestyle not a choice. Rabbi Brooks taught us that when you wake in the morning it is a gift and we should honor God with our first thoughts. Mode Ani is the prayer that is said every morning as soon as you reach consciousness.

- Hebrew: .מוֹדֶה (מוֹדָה) אֲנִי לְפָנֶיךָ מֶלֶךְ חַי וְקַיָּים
  שֶׁהֶחֱזַרְתָּ בִּי נִשְׁמָתִי בְּחֶמְלָה. רַבָּה אֱמוּנָתֶךְ:

  Transliteration: *Modeh ani lifanekha melekh ḥai v'kayam shehehezarta bi nishmahti b'ḥemlah, rabah emunatekha.*

  Translation: I offer thanks before you, living and eternal King, for You have mercifully restored my soul within me; Your faithfulness is great.

Mode Ani was very comforting for me because it helped me to shift my thinking from my fear of not making it to my Shepherd's faithfulness to walk with me through the painful journey that was ahead of me. Losing a loved one is not the end of the journey, it is just the beginning. The imagery of God as a Shepherd helps us to see God in a more compassionate, loving, guiding way. Mode Ani is taken from Lamentations 3:19-23 where it says, "*Remembering mine affliction and my misery, the wormwood and the gall. My soul hath them still in remembrance, and is humbled in me. This I recall to my mind, therefore have I hope. It is of the LORD's mercies that we are not consumed, because his compassions fail not. They are new every morning: great is thy faithfulness. The LORD is my portion, saith my soul; therefore will I hope in him."* Thirty-something years later Mode Ani still comforts me.

Grieving has a way of taking us through a myriad of emotions, thoughts, and questions. I am of the firm belief that it is perfectly normal to move through all of them. I currently serve as a Pediatric and Adult Chaplain for Delaware Hospice and as I walk with my patients and their families through their grieving process I see the myriad daily. As a Chaplain I understand that grieving is not just about death. It's about loss. The loss of what was, what is, and what could have been. I see how faith plays a major role in the lives of all that I encounter. My ministry is interfaith and the blessing in that is the opportunity to take God out of the box of "my way or the highway" thinking and experience God in a bigger more powerful way. As I think about my experience with grief I am reminded of Elizabeth Kubler Ross and her stages of grief. Her research has shown that as we experience loss, we all move through the five stages of grief: Denial, Anger, Bargaining, Depression, and Acceptance. When I reflect on my own story I can see where I shifted from one stage to the next. Although Kubler-Ross makes a good point I believe that our faith shifts with each phase as well.

Our faith is that which holds our hope, trust, and belief in God. Faith is the womb of all of our hopes and dreams. When our faith is shaken our lives are shaken. When I think about faith what comes to mind is water. Water moves in ways we never understand just like our faith does. The fluidity of water allows it to conform and transform to whatever the current reality is at the time. Water is a powerful force that can be calm at times and tumultuous at other times. Water does not cease to be water just because the conditions around it changes. Our faith must have that same fluidity to it. Our faith must remain intact regardless of the conditions around it. Fluidity is defined as a continuous, amorphous substance whose molecules move freely past one another and that has the tendency to assume the shape of its container. Faith is defined as a strong belief in something with no evidence and sometimes a strong belief in something even with evidence against it. To say that we must have fluid faith may sound strange for some people. The very idea of faith moving and not being steady may push some people beyond their comfort zone. Many of us have been taught that faith must be like a rock, unmovable and steadfast. That notion is taken from 1 Corinthians 15:58 (KJV) where it says, *"Therefore, my beloved brethren, be ye steadfast, unmovable, always abounding in the work of the Lord, forasmuch as ye know that your labour is not in vain in the Lord."* Unfortunately faith has been transposed into the text to mean the same thing as work. We must get to a place where we understand that we must release our faith from the jail of unmovability and release it to the realm of fluidity.

Our faith shifts as our grief shifts. I believe that we can look at the five stages of grief by Kubler Ross and associate our faith with each stage. We ask different faith questions as we move through the five stages of grief. My story was evident of that. When I was in denial about my son not having a heartbeat I asked, "God would not allow this to happen to me, right?" I was in the anger stage when the doctor told me for sure that my son died and I asked the question, "Why has God done this to me?" I moved to the bargaining stage when I secretly hoped that God would miraculously allow my baby to be born alive and I asked the question, "God if you let my son be born alive, I will….what do you require of me?" After my son was born and I did not get the miracle I expected I moved to the depression stage and I asked the question, "God where are You?" Finally, in the middle of the night when I was listening to *Jesus Is the Center of My Joy*, I moved to the final stage of acceptance where I asked the question, "God let your will be done, how do I move from here?"

With each question my faith became fluid like water. Symbolically my faith was like standing water when I was in the denial stage. It was not moving it was like a rock. I knew what I knew and nothing could change it. When I moved to the anger stage my faith was like running water. My faith was just a continuous drip of uncertainty. As I moved to the bargaining stage my faith became like rushing water. I was overwhelmed with the idea of a miracle. It had no basis in reality I was just all over the place. Eventually I moved to the depression stage and my faith was like flowing water. It was moving without my active participation. Finally I moved to the acceptance stage where my faith was like healing water. It was in this stage where I felt God's presence in my life and in my pain.

Psalms 23 stands as the official grieving scripture for many people. As I read that passage after the death of my son, Baby Corey, I was comforted. I found that passage to be reassuring that

God is with me even when my faith is moving due to the current condition of my life. Psalms 23 (KJV) says, *"The LORD is my shepherd; I shall not want. He maketh me to lie down in green pastures: he leadeth me beside the still waters. He restoreth my soul: he leadeth me in the paths of righteousness for his name's sake. Yea, though I walk through the valley of the shadow of death, I will fear no evil: for thou art with me; thy rod and thy staff they comfort me. Thou preparest a table before me in the presence of mine enemies: thou anointest my head with oil; my cup runneth over. Surely goodness and mercy shall follow me all the days of my life: and I will dwell in the house of the LORD forever."* Each line in this Psalm speaks to the fluidity of our faith.

This book was divinely inspired to help you shift from "rock faith" to "fluid faith" and Psalms 23 and Elizabeth Kubler-Ross's stages of grief is going to help us do just that. The book that you hold in your hands right now was created just for you. In your sadness, God is there. In your denial, God is there. In your anger, God is there. In your bargaining, God is there. In your depression, God is there. In your acceptance, God is there. At the end of each chapter is a prayer to begin your healing journey in that phase. I have given you space to write your own prayer as you seek God on your healing journey. Healing is a process. For some it may happen instantly or over-night. As you live with the loss of your loved one and attempt to find a new normal, healing happens. Give yourself grace and space to grieve. God is with you in and through your grief. Give yourself permission to move through the stages of grief at the time that makes sense to you. Every loss is not the same. Every grieving process has its own timeline. As you read this book allow the Holy Spirit to usher you through your grieving process in love, in peace, and in truth. Your Healing Journey Continues……………..

Chapter One
Standing Water

²He maketh me to lie down in green pastures: he leadeth me beside the still waters.

When I think about God and where I find myself in God what comes to mind is the womb. I say that because God designed the womb to be the dwelling place of life. Women have such an amazing journey through pregnancy. The first notion of being pregnant brings an overwhelming feeling of love. The baby may not even be the size of a pin head yet you love your baby, instantly. Fathers who desire to be fathers may experience love at first thought yet it is different for mothers because we have the distinct honor of being the dwelling place for this new little one. In the womb there is safety, in the womb there is warmth, in the womb there is sustenance, in the womb there is comfort. The absolutely amazing thing about the womb is that it grows with the baby not the other way around. The womb grows as the baby grows. God like the womb is our dwelling place. How we experience God grows as we grow. The womb does not cease to be in our lives. We are forever leaning and growing and God continues to be our safety, our warmth, our sustenance, and our comfort.

During the grieving process the womb of life may seem difficult. It reminds me of when I was pregnant with my first child. It was almost as if my son, K'Aelle, was trying to expand the womb on his own. He kicked, stretched, flipped, rolled around and I was so uncomfortable. I remember asking him what he was doing in there. He had no idea that what he was doing was making me uncomfortable. When we grieve, we kick, stretch, flip, and roll around. God, like the womb is there to hold us. The issue for some of us is that we want to break free from the confines of safety. If my son would have kicked his way out, he would not have survived he was not ready to leave the womb yet. God has some of us surrounded by the womb of Love and we are trying to get loose because we are in such pain. I am here to tell you, don't do it. God knows all about your pain, in time it will become bearable.

Standing Water is that place where our faith is like a rock. We refuse to be moved by what we see, what we hear, or what we feel. There is a time and a place for "rock faith". This is not that time. Faith is relative. I say that because it has to be birthed out of the current reality of the given situation. You cannot use the same faith for all situations. Our faith must be fluid enough to adjust while still remaining intact. I cannot use the same faith for every situation. If faith was a verb, an action, I could. Faith is a noun and that means it must be appropriated to a specific thing. Verbs can be used to describe various actions that can be interchangeable with many different things. The verb *flowing* can be used with water, wind, hair, music, etc. The noun mother can only be associated with a woman. You would never associate *mother* with a male because it just does not fit. As I walk with people through their grief journey I have found what I call a misappropriation of faith. Just like there is misappropriation of funds, there is misappropriation of faith. We habitually try to use blind faith, crazy faith, and unmovable faith in areas where they do not fit. Blind faith is found in Hebrews 11 (NLT) where it says,

"Faith is the confidence that what we hope for will actually happen; it gives us assurance about things we cannot see."

Crazy faith can be found in 1 Samuel 17:32-51(NLT) where we find the story of David killing Goliath.

"Don't worry about this Philistine," David told Saul. "I'll go fight him!" "Don't be ridiculous!" Saul replied. "There's no way you can fight this Philistine and possibly win! You're only a boy, and he's been a man of war since his youth." But David persisted. "I have been taking care of my father's sheep and goats," he said. "When a lion or a bear comes to steal a lamb from the flock, [35] I go after it with a club and rescue the lamb from its mouth. If the animal turns on me, I catch it by the jaw and club it to death. [36] I have done this to both lions and bears, and I'll do it to this pagan Philistine, too, for he has defied the armies of the living God! [37] The LORD who rescued me from the claws of the lion and the bear will rescue me from this Philistine!" Saul finally consented. "All right, go ahead," he said. "And may the LORD be with you!" Then Saul gave David his own armor—a bronze helmet and a coat of mail. David put it on, strapped the sword over it, and took a step or two to see what it was like, for he had never worn such things before. "I can't go in these," he protested to Saul. "I'm not used to them." So David took them off again. He picked up five smooth stones from a stream and put

them into his shepherd's bag. Then, armed only with his shepherd's staff and sling, he started across the valley to fight the Philistine. Goliath walked out toward David with his shield bearer ahead of him, sneering in contempt at this ruddy-faced boy. "Am I a dog," he roared at David, "that you come at me with a stick?" And he cursed David by the names of his gods. "Come over here, and I'll give your flesh to the birds and wild animals!" Goliath yelled. David replied to the Philistine, "You come to me with sword, spear, and javelin, but I come to you in the name of the LORD of Heaven's Armies—the God of the armies of Israel, whom you have defied. Today the LORD will conquer you, and I will kill you and cut off your head. And then I will give the dead bodies of your men to the birds and wild animals, and the whole world will know that there is a God in Israel! And everyone assembled here will know that the LORD rescues his people, but not with sword and spear. This is the LORD's battle, and he will give you to us!" As Goliath moved closer to attack, David quickly ran out to meet him. Reaching into his shepherd's bag and taking out a stone, he hurled it with his sling and hit the Philistine in the forehead. The stone sank in, and Goliath stumbled and fell face down on the ground. So David triumphed

23

over the Philistine with only a sling and a stone, for he had no sword. Then David ran over and pulled Goliath's sword from its sheath. David used it to kill him and cut off his head."

Unmovable faith can be found in Matthew 21:21 (KJV) where Jesus said,

Jesus answered and said unto them, Verily I say unto you, If ye have faith, and doubt not, ye shall not only do this which is done to the fig tree, but also if ye shall say unto this mountain, Be thou removed, and be thou cast into the sea; it shall be done."

Some would say that these three are the same faith. Let me show you how they are not. In Hebrews the faith is based on a future expectation, In 1 Samuel the faith is based on current confidence that the ability that God had given him would bring him the victory, and in Matthew Jesus is talking about believing for the manifestation of what you ask for. Each of these faiths is relative to the person doing the believing and the object of that belief. My faith is relative to my experience, my prayer life, and my relationship with God. I cannot use my Pastor's faith to deal with my challenges. My children cannot use my faith to trust God for themselves. When we misappropriate our faith we alter our healing process. How can I use crazy faith when my loved one is imminently dying and I have yet to say goodbye? How can I use blind faith when the doctor has told me that my son has died? How can I use unmovable faith when I have to decide whether to shift from quantity of life to quality of life so that I can help my loved one enjoy the days that they have left? I cannot tell a family to believe God for healing which for them is long life when cancer has spread to every area of the person's body. Yes we believe God, yes we know that God can do miraculous things yet we must be able to shift our thinking to accept when physical healing is no longer an option.

When I was in denial about my son not having a heartbeat I asked, "God would not allow this to happen to me, right?" In the standing water stage of our faith we tend to disbelieve our current reality. We emphatically deny the truth. It does not matter how big or how small the truth is. Refusing to believe the truth is our way of coping with the unbearable things in life. Does God know that we do that? absolutely. It is not a surprise to God that our faith alters our thinking. The surprise is for us because some of us have internalized a negative image of God. Love is not always the first

25

thing we think about when it comes to God. For some it is judgment, fear, and distance. Our assimilation of who God is must shift to a more loving image. The God that created us is a loving God, a compassionate God, and a God who cares about how we feel, what we think, and who we are.

Symbolically my faith was like standing water when I was in the denial stage. It was not moving it was like a rock. I knew what I knew and nothing could change it. I was in a state of shock. I couldn't accept the truth because it hurt too much. I believe that in this stage our faith is grounded in love yet uprooted in pain. I say that because faith is in us from birth. Babies have faith in their parents and only God could have given them that. How we experience our faith grows or remains stagnant based on how we are taught. We can learn to operate in faith in a positive way or a negative way. When we are faced with the loss of a loved one the ability to reason goes out of the window. Everything we have been taught seems to fade into the background of our pain. It is for this reason that we need to incorporate prayer. Prayer helps us to refocus, reframe, and reconnect. We must refocus our attention on what is true instead of what we have made ourselves believe. It is necessary to reframe, the ability to take the negative out of a situation and replace it with the positive, in order for us to move beyond the sting of the pain. Finally we must reconnect that which we disconnected, our communication with God.

"He maketh me to lie down in green pastures: he leadeth me beside the still waters" comes into play at this point. The notion that God would make us or put another way usher us, to *lie down in green pastures* means to me that God knows that in our pain we need guidance. *Lying down* can be seen as stilling ourselves and *green pastures* can be seen as being in a quiet peaceful place. *Leading us beside still waters* adds to stilling ourselves in a quiet peaceful place in that God's spirit of Love carries us to that place of calm. When we begin the grieving process we are unsure of what to do, what to expect, and how to move forward. I remember wondering how I was going to breathe again. It was if the news took my breath away. As you move from the denial stage your faith will move from it as well.

Allow this prayer to help you move:

Almighty and All Wise God, we thank you for your love, your grace, and your mercy. Right now I am asking you to help me face a hard truth. Help me to refocus my decisions, reframe my thinking, and reconnect my heart to you. This has to be one of the hardest things that I ever had to accept. Please help me to feel your love and your peace in my life right now. Amen.

MY PRAYER_____

_____

_____

_____

_____

_____

_____

_____

_____

_____

_____

_____

_____

_____

Chapter Two
Running Water

[3]He restoreth my soul: he leadeth me in the paths of righteousness for his name's sake.

Grieving has a way of eating away at the foundation of our faith. It reminds me of termites because the very nature of grief feeds off of our faith. Think about how you feel when you imagine losing someone. Immediately you begin to question what you believe you are able to withstand. Instinct tells you that it will never happen and doubt tells you that you won't make it. When I moved to the anger stage my faith was like running water. My faith was just a continuous drip of uncertainty. All I knew was that none of what I was going through was fair. I doubted my walk, I questioned my relationship with God, and I wavered in my faith. Anger surfaced because I was hurt. The thing that we miss about anger is that it is a surface emotion. When I say surface emotion I mean the emotion that presents itself while the deep seeded emotion remains hidden. Underneath anger is always hurt. If you think about it anger comes in response to someone that we are vulnerable to, transparent with, and connected to. Anger is not an issue with people who mean nothing to us because it does not matter. I was angry because I was so hurt that God would allow my son to die. I felt abandoned. I remember asking God, "Why didn't you warn me?" At that place in my life I believed that God and I had such a relationship that God would not throw me an emotional curve ball like that without warning.

I was in the anger stage when the doctor told me for sure that my son died and I asked the question, "Why has God done this to me?" The hurt that I felt was greater than any that I have ever experienced before in my life. As I lay there on the table rubbing what I had expected to be my health happy baby boy I thought about all that would never be. He would never meet me, he would never get to know his dad, his siblings, his family, and I would never know who he would have become. The anger stage can last a long time if we do not deal with the hurt issue. I always say, "*A hurt that has not been dealt with has no timeframe for healing.*" Many people have no idea why they are angry. I believe the trick of the adversary is to distract us with anger so that our hurt will not be healed. The Devil has no desire to see us whole and connected to God. The war is on and anger is the weapon. Look at the news anger is sustenance for the fuel of evil that is running rampant. The Devil knows that when the people of God are healed from their hurt and anger nothing will be able to disconnect us from God. Anger is a powerful negative force that we must get to know more about so that we can control it instead of it controlling us. Psychologists recognize three types of anger:

1. "Hasty and Sudden Anger" : the impulse for self-preservation which occurs when we are tormented or trapped
2. "Settled and Deliberate": reaction to perceived deliberate harm or unfair treatment of others
3. Dispositional: Character traits more than instincts or cognitions

Anger in Catholicism is counted as one of the seven deadly sins. In Hinduism, anger is equated with sorrow as a form of unrequited desire. Anger is considered to be packed with more evil power than desire. In Judaism, anger is a negative trait. Restraining oneself from anger is seen as noble and desirable. The Qur'an, the central religious text of Islam, attributes anger to prophets and believers and Muhammad's enemies. In general suppression of anger is deemed a praiseworthy quality and Muhammad is attributed to have said, "power resides not in being able to strike another, but in being able to keep the self under control when anger arises". Christians count anger as a negative emotion that is fueled by an undisciplined life. Anger is something to be controlled not the other way around. Anger in Buddhism is defined as: "being unable to bear the object, or the intention to cause harm to the object." Anger is seen as aversion with a stronger exaggeration, and is listed as one of the five hindrances. In Buddhism, the **five hindrances** (Pali: *pañca nīvaraṇāni*) are negative mental states that impede success with meditation (*jhāna* / *bhāvanā*) and lead away from enlightenment (nibbāna). These states are:

1. Sensual desire (*kāmacchanda*): Craving for pleasure to the senses.
2. Anger or ill-will (*byāpāda, vyāpāda*): Feelings of malice directed toward others.
3. Sloth-torpor or boredom (*thīna-middha*): Half-hearted action with little or no concentration.
4. Restlessness-worry (*uddhacca-kukkucca*): The inability to calm the mind.
5. Doubt (*vicikicchā*): Lack of conviction or trust.

The Buddhists believe that the mind controls the emotions and that when we get to a place of inner connectedness with ourselves we ultimately function better in the world. I was intrigued with the Buddhist concept of the Noble Eightfold Path. It intrigued me because the desire to cleanse the mind from the negative and replace it with the positive is what Jesus taught as He encountered so many along the way. Wrong thinking leads to wrong feeling which leads to wrong actions which leads to wrong living which leads to wrong loving. Love is who we are and what we are called to do and it all begins with right thinking. The Noble Eightfold Path is the fourth of the Buddha's Noble Truths (1. Life means suffering 2.The origin of suffering is attachment 3. The cessation of suffering is attainable 4. The path to the cessation of suffering).

The path has eight sections, each starting with the word "samyak" (Sanskrit, meaning "correctly", "properly", or "well", frequently translated into English as "right"), and presented in three groups known as the three higher trainings.

Prajñā is the wisdom that purifies the mind, allowing it to attain spiritual insight into the true nature of all things. It includes:

1. dṛṣṭi (ditthi): viewing reality as it is, not just as it appears to be;
2. saṃkalpa (sankappa): intention of renunciation, freedom and harmlessness.

Śīla is the ethics or morality, or abstention from unwholesome deeds. It includes:

3. vāc (vāca): speaking in a truthful and non-hurtful way;
4. karman (kammanta): acting in a non-harmful way;
5. ājīvana (ājīva): a non-harmful livelihood.

Samādhi is the mental discipline required to develop mastery over one's own mind. This is done through the practice of various contemplative and meditative practices, and includes:

6. vyāyāma (vāyāma): making an effort to improve;
7. smṛti (sati): awareness to see things for what they are with clear consciousness, being aware of the present reality within oneself, without any craving or aversion;
8. samādhi (samādhi): correct meditation or concentration, explained as the first four jhānas.

The practice of the Eightfold Path is understood in two ways, as requiring either simultaneous development (all eight items practiced in parallel), or as a progressive series of stages through which the practitioner moves, the culmination of one leading to the beginning of another. As we think about anger we must understand that anger is hard for many of us to get through on our own. We need some Divine intervention and prayer is the very thing that we need. Psalm 23 where it says, *"He restoreth my soul: he leadeth me in the paths of righteousness for his name's sake."* comes into play here. We need to be restored to our loving self because anger has taken over our thinking which has taken over how we live out our faith. When the Psalm talks about being led in the paths of righteousness we must understand that there is a process to come out of anger. The Buddhist practice of moving through the Noble Eightfold Path can help us as we pursue righteousness.

As a hospice Chaplain I have the pleasure of doing interfaith ministry and as I encounter different prayers I am moved by the universality of some of them. Buddhists have a wonderful concept of what it means to meditate through prayer. The purpose of Buddhist prayer is to awaken our inherent inner capacities of strength, compassion and wisdom rather than to petition external forces based on fear, idolizing, and worldly and/or heavenly gain. Buddhist prayer is a form of meditation; it is a practice of inner reconditioning. Buddhist prayer replaces the negative with the virtuous and points us to the blessings of life. Although it may be true that we all do not agree with everything we can agree that inner reconditioning is the pesticide to the seed of anger. One of the Buddhist prayers that I found comforting was the Universal Love Aspiration. I like it because the Bible says that God is love. It also says that God is a Spirit. It goes on to say that we were created in the image and likeness of God. With that understanding we can say that God is a Love Spirit and so are we. Love is who we are and what we do. Love has to be our motivating force and our guiding light.

Let this Love prayer help you shift your thinking.

Universal \Love Aspiration
Through the working of Great Compassion in their hearts,
May all beings have happiness and the causes of happiness,
May all be free from sorrow and the causes of sorrow;
May all never be separated from the sacred happiness, which is
sorrowless; And may all live in equanimity, Without too much
attachment and too much aversion; and live believing in the
equality of all that lives.

MY PRAYER_____

_____

_____

_____

_____

_____

_____

_____

_____

_____

_____

_____

_____

_____

_____

_____

_____

Chapter Three
Rushing Water

⁴Yea, though I walk through the valley of the shadow of death, I will fear no evil: for thou art with me; thy rod and thy staff they comfort me.

The grieving process brings an overwhelming sense of emotion. There are no words to describe how you truly feel when you are faced with the loss of someone you love very much. Unfortunately, I have come across some people who discredit the validity of experiencing grief. I have heard more times than I care to say that true believers don't grieve. My ears almost fell off when I heard it. People who say that believe that faith in God halts the grieving process and makes it non-existent. I totally disagree with that philosophy. There is no biblical text that affirms or confirms this way of thinking. Even Jesus acknowledged His grief. Right before Jesus went to the cross He stopped at the Garden to pray. The story unfolds in the Garden of Gethsemane right before Jesus was betrayed by Judas. Matthew 26: 36-46 (NLT) says, *"Then Jesus went with them to the olive grove called Gethsemane, and he* said, "Sit here while I go over there to pray." He took Peter and Zebedee's two sons, James and John, and he became anguished and distressed. He told them, "My soul is crushed with grief to the point of death. Stay here and keep watch with me." He went on a little farther and bowed with his face to the ground, praying, "My Father! If it is possible, let this cup of suffering be taken away from me. Yet I want your will to be done, not mine." Then he returned to the disciples and found them asleep. He said to Peter, "Couldn't you watch with me even one hour? Keep watch and pray, so that you will not give in to temptation. For the spirit is willing, but the body is weak!" Then Jesus left them a second time and prayed, "My Father! If this cup cannot be taken away unless I drink it, your will be done." When he returned to them again, he found them sleeping, for they couldn't keep their eyes open. So he went to pray a third time, saying the same things again. Then he came to the disciples and said, "Go ahead and sleep. Have your rest. But look—the time has come. The Son of Man is betrayed into the hands of sinners. Up, let's be going. Look, my betrayer is here!"

The story of Jesus praying in the garden is the perfect example of the grieving process. Jesus moved very quickly through all five stages. When Jesus said, *"My soul is crushed with grief to the point of death"*, He acknowledged that grief is a real emotion and that we all can experience it. Jesus was in denial when He asked God to take the cup of suffering because He already knew that He had to die for us to live. Jesus moved to the anger stage when he confronted his disciples about falling asleep. When Jesus said, *"My Father! If it is possible, let this cup of suffering be taken away from me Yet I want your will to be done, not mine"*, He was in the bargaining stage. Jesus moved to the depression stage when He said, *"My Father! If this cup cannot be taken away unless I drink it, your will be done."* After Jesus prayed the third time He accepted His call to be the salvation for all and submitted to God's will for His life.

I moved to the bargaining stage when I secretly hoped that God would miraculously allow my baby to be born alive and I asked the question, "God if you let my son be born alive, I will....what do you require of me?" I knew the real truth yet I wanted a different truth. I wanted to be released from the prison of grief just as Jesus did. I wanted to exchange my pain and at the same time I was willing to accept what God allowed. I was in a battle with myself. I knew the truth but I could not feel how it was going to set me free.

Sometimes our current reality is too painful to accept, too devastating to embrace, and too heartbreaking to experience. We make every attempt to escape the pain even bargain with God. As I moved to the bargaining stage my faith became like rushing water. I was overwhelmed with the idea of a miracle. It had no basis in reality I was just all over the place.

"Ye though I walk through the valley of the shadow of death" comes in at this point of our grief journey. As we think about what it means for us to walk through a valley suffering comes to mind. A valley experience comes with the feelings of abandonment, loneliness, and uncertainty. The question for many of us is will we keep walking. In the valley is the shadow of death and that means what appears to be real is not really real. Fluid faith has to kick in at this time. We need a faith that will move with us as we walk to shake our feelings of abandonment, loneliness, and uncertainty. As we walk the healing comes. It reminds me of the automatic doors at the hospital. The access is activated by motion. When you walk the door opens, when you stop the door remains closed. Our fluid faith works the same way. As we walk through the valley our access to God's

healing, calming presence is there. If we stop walking God does not cease to be there we cease to tap into God's presence.

Psalm 23 goes on to say, "*I will fear no evil for thou art with me. Thy rod and thy staff they comfort me.*" When we are in the bargaining stage fear kicks in more than any other stage. We experience the fear of losing control, the fear of losing our loved one, and the fear of losing ourselves. As human beings we have this misconception that we are human beings going through a spiritual experience. The truth of the matter is that we are spiritual beings going through a human experience. Genesis tells us that we were all created in the image and likeness of God and as I stated earlier God is Spirit. Jesus made that perfectly clear to the Samaritan woman at the well in John 4 when He declared that God is Spirit and they that worship God must worship in Spirit and in truth. Knowing that God is with us must be the turning point in our disconnection from God. When we talk to God we open our hearts to receive the guidance and love that the rod and the staff provide.

The rod conveys the concept of authority, of power, of discipline, of defense against danger, while the staff speaks of all that is loving and kind. The rod is there to turn us back to God when we stray. The staff draws us closer to God so that we can get the love and care that we need. Prayer is the way that we walk through the valley even in the midst of the shadows that scare us. Knowing God and feeling God are two different things. As you walk through your valley allow this Serenity Prayer by Reinhold Niebuhr to allow you to keep walking.

Your Healing Journey Continues.............

Allow this prayer to help you move:

God, grant me the serenity to accept the things I cannot change, the courage to change the things I can, and the wisdom to know the difference. Living one day at a time, enjoying one moment at a time; accepting hardship as a pathway to peace; taking, as Jesus did, this sinful world as it is, not as I would have it; trusting that You will make all things right if I surrender to Your will; so that I may be reasonably happy in this life and supremely happy with You forever in the next. Amen.

MY PRAYER_____

_____

_____

_____

_____

_____

_____

_____

_____

Chapter Four
Flowing Water

[5]Thou preparest a table before me in the presence of mine enemies: thou anointest my head with oil; my cup runneth over.

After my son was born and I did not get the miracle I expected I moved to the depression stage and I asked the question, "God where are You?" I felt so alone. I remember all the people who were in and out of my room trying to console me and it played like a silent black and white movie. I was so consumed with my grief that I saw them talking but could not really hear what they were saying. Have you ever been in a place where you felt like everything was moving in slow motion? Brokenness has a way of impeding the flow of our healing process. When we think about flowing water what comes to mind is tranquility however in our brokenness we don't feel tranquil, yet. It never ceases to amaze me how God can take our times of brokenness and use them to show us a better way.

In our brokenness we shift our faith from being self centered to being God centered. I say that because when we are broken our misguided notions, misdirected emotions, and misappropriation of our faith ceases to be. We have this misguided notion that we are alone and that no one else has ever felt the way that we do. The misdirected emotions are the ones that pull us away from our Shepherd. The emotional rollercoaster that we experience during the grieving process can consist of deep seeded hurt such as abandonment, helplessness, disappointment, and hopelessness. You may get to a point that you no longer want to live. The misappropriation of our faith comes in at this time because we on some level dismantle, disregard, and devalue our faith at this point. We make every attempt to dismantle the foundation of our faith, disregard the grace that is associated with our faith, and devalue the changing power in our faith in our attempt to walk away from our Shepherd because we feel that our Shepherd has walked away from us. We are in a place called spiritual depression. It is in this place that we have nowhere to go but up. Our hearts are broken and our spirits are in distress. We have made every attempt to isolate ourselves from other people and from God. We have this idea that our broken heart is separate from our spiritual journey when the truth is that the state of our heart is directly connected with the state of our spirit.

Proverbs 15:13 confirms the fact that our heart and our spirit are connected. When you read the Proverb in different versions it helps to confirm my point in a better way. The King James Version says, "*A merry heart maketh a **cheerful countenance**: but by sorrow of the heart the **spirit is broken**"*. The King James helps us to see a direct connection between the countenance and the state of the spirit. The Message Bible says, "*A cheerful heart **brings a smile** to your face; a sad heart **makes it hard to get through the day**.*" The Message Bible helps us to see what our response to emotional distress looks like. The Good News Bible says, "*When people are happy, they **smile**, but when they are sad, they **look depressed**.*" This version helps us to see how our emotional experiences can alter our emotional state from happiness to depression. The New Living Translation says, "*A glad heart makes a **happy** face; a broken heart **crushes** the spirit.*" This is the version that really helps us to see that our brokenness can lead to spiritual depression. The crushed spirit has nothing to do with our faith. Faith at this point is on auto pilot. I say that because we live, move, and have our being in the residue of who God has been in our lives. When I was deep in my grief my faith was like flowing water. It was moving without my active participation. The strength that I had to fight was gone. The mindset to press on was gone. What I had was brokenness. I was at a place where all I could do was rely on God to help me through because I just could not do it on my own.

Psalm 23 played a major part in this stage of my grief. It says, *"Thou prepares a table before me in the presence of mine enemies"*. Now imagine sitting at a prepared table in front of your enemies. Chaos all around and there sits a table for you. Well what is on the table? Why is it in the presence of your enemies? I believe 2 Corinthians 4 will help us understand this a little better. We will use four different versions of 2 Corinthians 4:8-9 to help explain this point. The King James says, *"We are troubled on every side, yet not distressed; we are perplexed, but not in despair; Persecuted,* ***but not forsaken****; cast down, but not destroyed."* King James helps us to see that the *table* sits to be our reassurance that God is with us throughout our troubles. The Good News says, *"We are often troubled, but not crushed;* ***sometimes in doubt****, but never in despair; there are many enemies, but* ***we are never without a friend; and***

50

though badly hurt at times, we are not destroyed." The Good News helps us to see that even in our doubt and in our brokenness God has not left us. The Message Bible says, "*We've been surrounded and battered by troubles, but we're not demoralized; we're not sure what to do, but* **we know that God knows what to do; we've been spiritually terrorized**, *but God hasn't left our side; we've been thrown down, but we haven't broken.*" The wonderful thing about the Message is that it describes our uncertainty and our spiritual distress yet we have full confidence that God knows what God is doing. Finally, the New Living says, "*We are pressed on every side,* **but we still have room to move**. *We are often in much trouble, but we never give up. People make it hard for us, but we are not left alone. We are knocked down, but we are not destroyed.*" The New Living seals the deal. It shares the amazing fact that even at the table in the midst of our enemies **we still have room to move**." When I read that verse I immediately thought about flowing water and I understood that God has a way of ushering us to a better place whether we are active participants or not. Faith is deep seeded and even when we don't know how to tap into it and activate it God recognizes that it is there and moves on our behalf. The Psalm goes

51

on to say, *"Thou anointest my head with oil, my cup runneth over."*
God knows our faith barometer and anoints us to compensate for
what is lacking. The anointing is God's purpose poured on us with
power. God taps into the part of us that is connected to God. When
our faith is like flowing water it moves as God moves.

Think about a child when they are learning to walk. The
parent guides them throughout the journey. Even when they get
discouraged and want to give up the parent takes the child by the
hand and leads the child until the child can walk on their own. The
ability to walk was always there just as our faith was always there
when we thought we could no longer walk. God put the table there
and anointed you to sustain you and for you to know that you are
never alone.

When I think about being anointed and my cup running over
singing comes to mind. I have found that singing helps me to reverse
my attempts to disconnect. There is something about music that
sweetly ushers our spirit to a place of worship. When we allow the
fluidity of our faith to move us to a place of worship those things
which held us hostage lose their power over us. There is a wonderful

hymn called *Draw Me Nearer* that says, "I am thine O Lord and I heard your voice and it told thy love to me. But I long to rise in the arms of faith and be closer drawn to thee" That song makes it very clear that God's love draws us even when we attempt to disconnect. Isn't it amazing that Love actively pursues us no matter where we are, no matter what we think, no matter how we feel, and no matter where our faith is at that time. The song says I long to rise in the arms of faith and that means to me that God loves us so much that we can reach up to God as far as we can and God will reach down the carry us the rest of the way. When our faith is like flowing water God steps in to protect us from ourselves. I say that because in our attempt to disconnect from our Shepherd we have no idea what awaits us outside of the sheepfold. Danger is awaiting us for the enemy comes to steal, kill, and destroy. Let God help you through this stage and I guarantee you that your life will never be the same.

There is a story in John 5 that will help those who are stuck in the depression stage move to the final stage of acceptance. The story unfolds in John 5 and says, *"After this there was a feast of the Jews; and Jesus went up to Jerusalem. Now there is at Jerusalem by the sheep market a pool, which is called in the Hebrew tongue*

Bethesda, having five porches. In these lay a great multitude of impotent folk, of blind, halt, withered, waiting for the moving of the water. For an angel went down at a certain season into the pool, and troubled the water: whosoever then first after the troubling of the water stepped in was made whole of whatsoever disease he had. And a certain man was there, which had an infirmity thirty and eight years. When Jesus saw him lie, and knew that he had been now a long time in that case, he saith unto him, Wilt thou be made whole?" This story meets us right where we are. The season is here, the angel has descended, the water has been troubled, the question for you is will you be made whole?

Your Healing Journey Continues..............

Let this prayer move you to wholeness.

Jehovah Rapha, God my healer thank you for meeting me right where I am. Thank you for loving me even when I have not loved myself. Thank you for being faithful even when I am not faithful. Help me God to move from my brokenness. I need your help, I need your guidance, and I need your healing power in my life. Amen

MY PRAYER_____

_____

_____

_____

_____

_____

_____

_____

_____

_____

_____

_____

Chapter Five
Healing Water

⁶Surely goodness and mercy shall follow me all the days of my life: and I will dwell in the house of the LORD forever.

In the middle of the night when I was listening to *Jesus Is the Center of My Joy*, I moved to the final stage of acceptance where I asked the question, "God let your will be done, how do I move on from here?" Although I had accepted that my son was gone and I needed to move on I still did not know how. My heart had to catch up with my mind. What do you mean, I am glad you asked. I mean that my mind had reframed, replaced the positive with the negative, what I was experiencing yet my heart still needed some mending. I was reminded of a story in Ezekiel.

Ezekiel 47:1-10 (NKJV) says, " *Then he brought me back to the door of the temple; and there was water, flowing from under the threshold of the temple toward the east, for the front of the temple faced east; the water was flowing from under the right side of the temple, south of the altar. He brought me out by way of the north gate, and led me around on the outside to the outer gateway that faces east; and there was water, running out on the right side. And when the man went out to the east with the line in his hand, he measured one thousand cubits, and he brought me through the waters; the water came up to my ankles. Again he measured one thousand and brought me through the waters; the water came up to my knees. Again he measured one thousand and brought me through; the water came up to my waist. Again he measured one thousand, and it was a river that I could not cross; for the water was too deep, water in which one must swim, a river that could not be crossed. He said to me, "Son of man, have you seen this?" Then he brought me and returned me to the bank of the river. When I returned, there, along the bank of the river, were very many trees on one side and the other. Then he said to me: "This water flows toward the eastern region, goes down into the valley, and enters the sea. When it reaches the sea, its waters are healed. "And it shall be that every living thing that moves, wherever the rivers go, will live."*

In Ezekiel the water represented the healing that I needed and the place where the water reaches was the level of hurt that my heart felt. Some of us are hurt to our ankles and can recover easily. Some of us are hurt to our knees and can recover with a little help. Some of us are hurt up to our waist and can recover with a lot of help. While some of us have been hurt so bad that the waters are too deep and we cannot cross them. It is in this place of the valley that we find ourselves in desperate need of the healing waters. When our hurt is so deep that we cannot cross we understand that we need Divine intervention. That is exactly where I found myself. I needed God to step out of time into my time right on time to be a present help for me. When I listened to the song, *Jesus Is the Center of My Joy,* amazingly my hurt flowed out of me in my tears. Crying is a wonderful way to cleanse the soul. Many of us have been told that it is not okay to cry, well beloved Jesus wept after Lazarus died and He also wept over Jerusalem. If Jesus cried so can we.

When I finally moved to the acceptance stage where my faith was like healing water, I felt God's presence in my life and in my pain. I reflected on Psalm 23 where it said, *"Surely goodness and mercy shall follow me all the days of my life."* When I think about God's goodness I can't help but to smile. When I look back over my life and I think things over I know God has kept me my whole life.

I understand that there is nothing too hard for God and just like the song says, I have come this far by faith leaning on the Lord. I had to realize that I came too far to turn back now. When I thought about the mercy of God I had to recall the mercy that God showed my son. Baby Corey would have suffered and I asked God for a healthy happy baby and even though it did not come that way I thought it would however I got what I asked for. The healing water of God comes at a time when we need it the most. Our hearts must be ready to receive God's healing in our lives.

As we move to the acceptance stage our faith shifts out of auto pilot. We become active participants in our faith journey. That which attempted to hold us hostage has been overcome. The things in our lives that made us believe that we could not make it have been silenced. We move to a place where we can breathe again. The shock of the loss, the sting of the loss, the disbelief of the loss, and the overwhelming pain of the loss is now in the recesses of our minds. Now this does not mean that all of them cannot and will not be triggered by various things. The good news is that the healing that we have received from God will keep us. I am continually amazed at how God took my tears of sorrow and changed them to tears of joy. Isaiah 61:3 confirms this where it says, *"To appoint unto them that mourn in Zion, to give unto them **beauty for ashes**, the **oil of joy for mourning**, the **garment of praise for the spirit of heaviness;** that they might be called trees of righteousness, the planting of the LORD, that he might be glorified."* Every time I hear *Jesus is the Center of My Joy* I smile and think about my little baby that is beauty for ashes. Every year on his birthday God gives me a special anointing not to go back to my time of depression that's my oil for mourning. Whenever I have to share my story God ushers me into a place of praise for making it through that is my garment of praise for the spirit of heaviness. God has a way of making a way out of no way to get us out of the way.

Healing water comes right when we need it. As our faith moves with fluidity the spirit of Love does as well. God knows what we need before we even need it or even know we need it. As you allow the healing waters to cover you know that the process is necessary. Psalms 23 closes with, *"And I will dwell in the house of the Lord forever"* and the only way we can do that is if we have complete trust in God. Trials are going to come, trouble will come, hurt and pain will come, and loss will as well. As we hold on to God's unchanging hand we will be forever mindful that there are some things we will never get over, YET WE GET THROUGH.

Your Healing Journey Continues..............

Allow this prayer to help you move:

Gracious and Loving God thank you for being Love. Thank you for being patient with me. Thank you for saving me from myself. Thank you for never leaving me alone. Today I give myself to you so that you can heal my brokenness. In my doubt, in my wavering faith, in my pain I step into the healing waters knowing that my time of healing is now. Amen

MY PRAYER_____

_____

_____
_____
_____
_____
_____
_____
_____
_____
_____
_____
_____
_____
_____
_____
_____
_____

FOR ADDITIONAL MEDIA RESOURCES

OR TO SCHEDULE THE AUTHOR FOR

SPEAKING ENGAGEMENTS OR SPECIAL EVENTS,

CONTACT

REV. DR. A'SHELLARIEN LANG

267-779-1475

WWW.DESAKAJOSFLO.COM

Made in the USA
Middletown, DE
22 January 2022

59406277R00036